NATURAL REMEDIES AND CURE FOR CANCER

How to Cure and Prevent Cancer Naturally

DR. ARTHUR MYLES

TABLE OF CONTENTS

INTRODUCTION

Cancer is a complex and multifaceted disease that affects millions of people worldwide. The journey through cancer treatment can be physically, emotionally, and mentally challenging. While conventional treatments such as chemotherapy, radiation, and surgery are the cornerstone of cancer care, many patients and caregivers explore complementary and alternative therapies, including natural remedies, to support the healing process and improve quality of life.

Natural remedies encompass a wide range of practices and substances, from dietary changes and herbal supplements to mind-body practices like meditation and yoga. These approaches are often sought to alleviate side effects of conventional treatments, enhance overall well-being, and, in some cases, potentially contribute to the fight against cancer.

Natural remedies are generally used as complementary treatments, meaning they are integrated with, rather than replace, standard medical care. The goal is to create a holistic approach to cancer treatment that supports the body, mind, and spirit.

It is essential to understand that natural remedies should not be seen as substitutes for conventional cancer therapies. While some natural remedies have shown promise in studies, they are not a cure for cancer. The effectiveness of natural remedies can vary depending on the type of cancer, the stage of the disease, and individual patient factors.

Integrating natural remedies with conventional treatments requires careful consideration and collaboration with healthcare providers. This ensures that any natural approach taken does not interfere with standard treatments or cause adverse effects. For instance, certain herbal supplements may interact with chemotherapy drugs, reducing their efficacy or increasing side effects.

Before incorporating any natural remedy into a cancer care plan, it is crucial to consult with a healthcare professional, ideally one who is knowledgeable in both conventional oncology and integrative medicine. This collaboration allows for personalized recommendations that take into account the patient's specific medical condition, treatment plan, and overall health.

Healthcare providers can help guide decisions regarding the use of natural remedies, ensuring they are safe, effective, and appropriate. They can also monitor for potential interactions and adjust treatment plans as needed.

Natural remedies can play a valuable role in supporting cancer treatment, improving quality of life, and addressing the holistic needs of patients. However, they must be used thoughtfully and in conjunction with conventional medical care. By working closely with healthcare professionals, patients can explore natural remedies in a safe and informed manner, contributing to a comprehensive and personalized approach to cancer care.

CHAPTER 1
History of Cancer

Cancer, as a disease, has a history that stretches back thousands of years. Its understanding, classification, and treatment have evolved significantly over time, shaped by advancements in science, medicine, and technology. The journey from ancient times to the modern era reveals how perceptions of cancer have changed and how humanity has sought to combat this formidable disease.

Ancient Times: The Earliest Records

The earliest known descriptions of cancer date back to ancient Egypt, around 3000 BCE. The Edwin Smith Papyrus, an ancient Egyptian medical text, describes cases of tumors or ulcers of the breast, treated by cauterization. The document explicitly states that there is no known treatment for the condition, highlighting the challenges faced by ancient physicians.

The term "cancer" itself comes from the Greek word "karkinos," meaning crab, coined by the Greek physician Hippocrates (460–370 BCE). He used the term to describe tumors because the projections from some tumors resembled the claws of a crab. Hippocrates also categorized cancers as either "carcinos" or "carcinoma" based on their physical characteristics. His work laid the foundation for the future understanding of cancer, though treatment options at the time were limited to surgical removal when possible.

Middle Ages: Stagnation and Superstition

During the Middle Ages, the understanding of cancer did not advance significantly. The disease was often seen through a lens of superstition and religious belief. Many believed that cancer was a punishment from the gods or a result of an imbalance of the body's humors, a theory popularized by Hippocrates and later Galen, another prominent Greek physician. Treatments were rudimentary and often harmful, including bloodletting, purging, and the use of various herbs and potions.

Renaissance to the 18th Century: Emerging Understanding

The Renaissance period brought renewed interest in science and medicine, leading to more systematic studies of diseases, including cancer. Autopsies became more common, allowing physicians to study tumors in greater detail. In the 16th century, the Swiss physician Paracelsus proposed that cancer was not caused by an imbalance of humors but by external factors, although his ideas were not widely accepted at the time.

In the 18th century, the Scottish surgeon John Hunter made significant contributions to cancer surgery, advocating for the surgical removal of tumors that were localized and not spread to other parts of the body. This was a major step forward in the treatment of cancer, though the concept of metastasis (the spread of cancer) was not yet fully understood.

19th Century: The Birth of Modern Oncology

The 19th century saw dramatic advancements in medical science, including the development of anesthesia and antiseptic techniques, which made more extensive and safer cancer surgeries possible. Rudolf Virchow, a German physician, and pathologist, advanced the understanding of cancer by proposing that it originated from normal cells that had undergone abnormal changes. His work laid the groundwork for the field of cellular pathology.

Around the same time, the development of the microscope allowed for more detailed examination of cancerous tissues, leading to better classification and understanding of different types of cancer. The recognition of cancer as a group of related diseases, rather than a single disease, was a crucial step in developing more targeted treatments.

20th Century: The Era of Scientific Breakthroughs

The 20th century marked a turning point in cancer research and treatment. The discovery of X-rays by

Wilhelm Roentgen in 1895 and the subsequent development of radiation therapy provided a new tool for treating cancer. This was followed by the introduction of chemotherapy in the 1940s, beginning with the use of nitrogen mustard, a chemical weapon repurposed for medical use. The success of chemotherapy in treating certain cancers, like leukemia, sparked a wave of research into other chemical compounds that could target cancer cells.

The 1950s and 1960s saw the establishment of cancer research institutions and the beginning of large-scale clinical trials, which helped standardize treatments and improve patient outcomes. The understanding of genetics and molecular biology also advanced during this period, leading to the discovery of oncogenes and tumor suppressor genes, which play a critical role in cancer development.

21st Century: Precision Medicine and Beyond
In the 21st century, the focus of cancer treatment has shifted towards precision medicine, which tailors treatment to the individual characteristics of each patient's cancer. Advances in genetic sequencing and molecular profiling have enabled the development of targeted therapies that attack specific cancer mutations while sparing healthy cells. Immunotherapy, which harnesses the body's immune system to fight cancer, has also emerged as a powerful treatment option, particularly for

cancers that were previously considered untreatable.

The advent of personalized medicine, along with improvements in early detection and prevention, has led to significant improvements in survival rates for many types of cancer. Research continues to explore new frontiers, including the potential of artificial intelligence, nanotechnology, and gene editing in cancer treatment.

The history of cancer is a testament to human perseverance in the face of one of nature's most formidable challenges. From ancient Egypt to the cutting-edge research of today, the understanding and treatment of cancer have evolved dramatically. While the battle against cancer is ongoing, the progress made thus far provides hope for continued advancements in the quest to prevent, treat, and ultimately cure this disease.

Types of Cancer
Cancer is a complex group of diseases characterized by the uncontrolled growth and spread of abnormal cells. There are many types of cancer, each classified based on the location in the body where it originates, the type of cell involved, and the pattern of growth. Understanding the different types of cancer can help in recognizing symptoms, determining treatment options, and providing appropriate care.

Carcinomas

Carcinomas are cancers that originate in the epithelial cells, which line the surfaces and cavities of the body. They are the most common type of cancer.

Adenocarcinoma: Develops in glandular tissues, such as the breast, prostate, or colon.
Squamous Cell Carcinoma: Originates in the squamous cells lining the skin or mucous membranes, commonly found in the lungs, mouth, and skin.
Basal Cell Carcinoma: Typically arises in the basal cells of the skin and is often associated with sun exposure.

Sarcomas

Sarcomas are cancers that arise from connective tissues, such as bones, muscles, fat, and cartilage.

Osteosarcoma: Affects bone tissue and is most common in adolescents and young adults.
Chondrosarcoma: Develops in cartilage tissue and can occur in any cartilage-containing area.
Liposarcoma: Originates in fat cells and can occur in various body parts.

Leukemias

Leukemias are cancers of the blood and bone marrow characterized by the overproduction of abnormal white blood cells.

Acute Lymphoblastic Leukemia (ALL): Affects immature lymphocytes and progresses rapidly.
Acute Myeloid Leukemia (AML): Involves abnormal myeloid cells and progresses quickly.
Chronic Lymphocytic Leukemia (CLL): Affects mature lymphocytes and progresses slowly.
Chronic Myeloid Leukemia (CML): Involves abnormal myeloid cells and progresses over time.

Lymphomas

Lymphomas are cancers of the lymphatic system, which is part of the body's immune system.

Hodgkin Lymphoma: Characterized by the presence of Reed-Sternberg cells and typically affects lymph nodes.
Non-Hodgkin Lymphoma: Includes various subtypes, such as B-cell and T-cell lymphomas, and can affect lymph nodes and other organs.

Myelomas

Myelomas are cancers that arise from plasma cells, a type of white blood cell found in the bone marrow.

Multiple Myeloma: Involves the abnormal proliferation of plasma cells in the bone marrow, leading to bone damage and kidney problems.

Melanomas

Melanomas are cancers that develop from melanocytes, the cells responsible for producing pigment in the skin.

Cutaneous Melanoma: Occurs in the skin and is often linked to sun exposure.
Ocular Melanoma: Develops in the eye and is less common than cutaneous melanoma.

Neuroendocrine Tumors

Neuroendocrine tumors originate from cells that release hormones into the bloodstream in response to nerve signals.

Carcinoid Tumor: A type of neuroendocrine tumor typically found in the gastrointestinal tract or lungs.
Pancreatic Neuroendocrine Tumor: Arises in the pancreas and may produce excess hormones.

Germ Cell Tumors

Germ cell tumors develop from germ cells, which are involved in reproduction.

Testicular Germ Cell Tumor: Includes seminomas and non-seminomas, affecting the testicles.

Ovarian Germ Cell Tumor: Includes various subtypes, such as dysgerminomas and teratomas, affecting the ovaries.

Brain and Spinal Cord Tumors
These tumors arise in the central nervous system and can be either primary (originating in the brain or spinal cord) or secondary (metastatic, originating elsewhere and spreading to the brain or spinal cord).

Gliomas: Tumors that originate from glial cells, including astrocytomas and oligodendrogliomas.
Meningiomas: Arise from the meninges, the protective layers covering the brain and spinal cord.
Medulloblastomas: Common in children and originate in the cerebellum.

Rare and Other Cancers
There are several rare types of cancer that do not fit neatly into the categories above.

Pleomorphic Sarcoma: A rare and aggressive form of sarcoma.
Chordoma: A rare bone cancer that occurs in the spine or skull base.

The diversity of cancer types reflects the complexity of the disease, with each type having its own characteristics, treatment approaches, and prognosis. Accurate diagnosis and classification are crucial for determining the most effective treatment strategies and providing personalized care. Understanding the specific type of cancer can help patients, families, and healthcare providers work together to manage the disease and support overall health and well-being.

CHAPTER 2
Diet and Nutrition

Diet and nutrition play a crucial role in overall health and well-being, and they are particularly important in the context of cancer. While no specific diet can cure cancer, a well-balanced and nutritious diet can support the body's immune system, improve the effectiveness of conventional treatments, and help manage side effects. Additionally, certain foods and nutrients have been studied for their potential to reduce cancer risk or inhibit the growth of cancer cells.

Antioxidant-Rich Foods

Antioxidants are compounds that help protect the body from oxidative stress, which can damage cells and contribute to cancer development. Incorporating antioxidant-rich foods into the diet can support the body's natural defenses against cancer.

Berries: Blueberries, strawberries, raspberries, and blackberries are rich in vitamins, minerals, and phytochemicals like anthocyanins, which have strong antioxidant properties.

Leafy Greens: Spinach, kale, and other dark leafy greens are packed with vitamins A, C, and E, along with other antioxidants that may help protect cells from damage.

Nuts and Seeds: Almonds, walnuts, chia seeds, and flaxseeds provide a good source of antioxidants, healthy fats, and fiber, contributing to overall health.

Turmeric (Curcumin)

Turmeric is a spice commonly used in Indian cuisine, and it contains an active compound called curcumin, which has been studied for its anti-inflammatory and anti-cancer properties. Curcumin may help slow the growth of certain types of cancer cells and enhance the effectiveness of chemotherapy. It is best absorbed when consumed with black pepper and fat, such as olive oil or coconut oil.

Usage: Turmeric can be added to a variety of dishes, including soups, stews, curries, and smoothies. Curcumin supplements are also available, but should be used under the guidance of a healthcare provider.

Green Tea

Green tea is rich in polyphenols, particularly catechins like epigallocatechin gallate (EGCG), which have been shown to have anti-cancer properties. Studies suggest that green tea may help inhibit the growth of cancer cells and reduce the risk of developing certain types of cancer, such as breast, prostate, and colorectal cancer.

Consumption: Drinking 2-3 cups of green tea daily may provide health benefits. It can be enjoyed hot or cold and can be flavored with lemon or honey.

Garlic and Onions

Garlic and onions are members of the allium family and contain sulfur compounds that have been linked to anti-cancer effects. These compounds may help detoxify carcinogens, inhibit cancer cell growth, and reduce inflammation. Regular consumption of garlic and onions has been associated with a reduced risk of cancers, particularly stomach and colorectal cancers.

Incorporation: Garlic and onions can be added to a wide range of dishes, including salads, sauces, soups, and stir-fries. For maximum benefit, garlic should be chopped or crushed and allowed to sit for a few minutes before cooking.

Cruciferous Vegetables

Cruciferous vegetables, such as broccoli, cauliflower, Brussels sprouts, and cabbage, contain glucosinolates, which are broken down into active compounds like sulforaphane and indole-3-carbinol. These compounds have been studied for their ability to detoxify carcinogens, protect DNA from damage, and inhibit the growth of cancer cells.

Dietary Tips: Aim to include cruciferous vegetables in your diet several times a week. They can be steamed, roasted, or added to salads and stir-fries.

Healthy Fats

Incorporating healthy fats into the diet is important for maintaining energy levels and supporting the absorption of fat-soluble vitamins. Omega-3 fatty acids, found in fatty fish like salmon, mackerel, and sardines, as well as in flaxseeds and walnuts, have anti-inflammatory properties and may reduce the risk of cancer.

Cooking Advice: Use olive oil or avocado oil for cooking and salad dressings. Include fatty fish in your diet at least twice a week, and snack on nuts and seeds.

Fiber-Rich Foods

A diet high in fiber supports digestive health and can help reduce the risk of colorectal cancer. Fiber-rich foods also promote a healthy gut microbiome, which is increasingly recognized as important for overall health and immunity.

Sources: Whole grains, legumes, fruits, vegetables, and seeds are excellent sources of dietary fiber. Aim for at least 25-30 grams of fiber per day.

Diet and nutrition are powerful tools in supporting cancer treatment and prevention. By focusing on a diet rich in antioxidants, anti-inflammatory foods, and healthy fats, and by minimizing processed and high-sugar foods, individuals can enhance their body's natural defenses and improve their overall health. However, it's important to remember that diet is just one aspect of cancer care and should be part of a comprehensive approach that includes medical treatment, regular exercise, and stress management.

CHAPTER 3

Herbal Remedies

Herbal remedies have been used for centuries in various cultures to promote health and treat illness. In the context of cancer, some herbs are believed to support the immune system, reduce treatment side effects, and possibly inhibit cancer cell growth. However, the efficacy and safety of these remedies can vary, and they should be used in conjunction with, not as a replacement for, conventional cancer treatments. Always consult with a healthcare provider before incorporating herbal remedies into your cancer care plan.

Milk Thistle

Milk thistle (Silybum marianum) is a flowering herb that has been used for centuries to support liver health. The active compound in milk thistle, silymarin, is a potent antioxidant and anti-inflammatory agent. It is believed to protect the liver from toxins and may have a role in supporting the liver during chemotherapy or other cancer treatments that can be taxing on the liver.

Potential Benefits: Some studies suggest that silymarin may help reduce liver toxicity and improve liver function in patients undergoing chemotherapy. There is also interest in its potential anti-cancer properties, although more research is needed.

Usage: Milk thistle is available as a supplement in capsules, tablets, or liquid extracts. Dosages vary, so it's important to follow the guidance of a healthcare provider.

Astragalus

Astragalus (Astragalus membranaceus) is a traditional Chinese herb that has been used to strengthen the immune system and support overall vitality. It is known for its adaptogenic properties, meaning it helps the body adapt to stress. In cancer care, astragalus is often used to boost immune function, especially in patients undergoing chemotherapy or radiation therapy.

Potential Benefits: Some studies suggest that astragalus may enhance the effectiveness of chemotherapy, improve survival rates, and reduce treatment-related side effects like fatigue and immunosuppression. It is also being studied for its potential to inhibit tumor growth.

Usage: Astragalus can be consumed as a tea, tincture, or supplement. It is often combined with other herbs in traditional Chinese medicine formulas. Dosage should be determined by a qualified healthcare provider.

Essiac Tea

Essiac tea is an herbal formula that originated in Canada and is named after its creator, nurse Rene Caisse (Essiac is Caisse spelled backward). The formula typically includes burdock root, sheep sorrel, slippery elm bark, and Indian rhubarb root. Essiac tea has been promoted as a natural cancer treatment, although scientific evidence supporting its efficacy is limited.

Potential Benefits: Proponents of Essiac tea claim it supports detoxification, boosts the immune system, and helps fight cancer. However, clinical studies on Essiac tea are inconclusive, and it should not be used as a primary treatment for cancer.

Usage: Essiac tea is usually consumed as a brewed tea. It's important to follow specific preparation instructions and consult with a healthcare provider before use, as some of the ingredients may interact with conventional cancer treatments.

Turmeric (Curcumin)

Turmeric, known for its bright yellow color, is widely used as a spice and medicinal herb. Curcumin, the active compound in turmeric, has been extensively studied for its anti-inflammatory and anti-cancer properties. It is believed to inhibit cancer cell growth, reduce inflammation, and enhance the effectiveness of certain chemotherapy drugs.

Potential Benefits: Curcumin has been shown to interfere with cancer cell signaling pathways, potentially slowing the growth of cancer cells and making them more susceptible to treatment. It may also reduce inflammation and oxidative stress in the body.

Usage: Turmeric can be used in cooking or taken as a supplement. For cancer support, curcumin supplements with enhanced bioavailability are often recommended. It should be taken with black pepper (piperine) and fat to improve absorption.

Ginger

Ginger (Zingiber officinale) is a popular herbal remedy known for its anti-nausea and anti-inflammatory properties. It is commonly used to alleviate nausea and vomiting associated with chemotherapy. Additionally, ginger has antioxidant and anti-cancer properties that may help protect against certain types of cancer.

Potential Benefits: Ginger may help reduce chemotherapy-induced nausea and vomiting. It also contains compounds like gingerol and shogaol, which have shown potential in inhibiting cancer cell growth in laboratory studies.

Usage: Ginger can be consumed fresh, as a tea, or in supplement form. It can also be added to foods and beverages. For nausea relief, ginger tea or ginger candies are commonly used.

Green Tea

Green tea is rich in polyphenols, particularly catechins like epigallocatechin gallate (EGCG), which have powerful antioxidant and anti-cancer properties. Studies suggest that green tea may help prevent certain types of cancer and support the body's natural defenses against cancer cells.

Potential Benefits: Green tea may reduce the risk of developing cancers such as breast, prostate, and colorectal cancer. It is also believed to enhance the effectiveness of certain cancer treatments and support overall health.

Usage: Drinking 2-3 cups of green tea daily can provide health benefits. Green tea extracts are also available in supplement form, but it's important to consult a healthcare provider before use.

Mistletoe

Mistletoe (Viscum album) is a plant used in traditional European medicine for various ailments, including cancer. Mistletoe extracts are used in some European countries as part of integrative cancer treatment. It is believed to stimulate the immune system, improve quality of life, and potentially slow tumor growth.

Potential Benefits: Some studies suggest that mistletoe therapy may improve survival rates, enhance quality of life, and reduce the side effects of chemotherapy and radiation therapy. However, more research is needed to confirm these effects.

Usage: Mistletoe therapy is usually administered through injections under the skin. It should only be used under the supervision of a healthcare provider experienced in its use.

Herbal remedies offer a complementary approach to cancer care, potentially helping to manage symptoms, reduce side effects, and support overall well-being. However, it is essential to approach these remedies with caution, as they can interact with conventional treatments and may not be appropriate for all individuals. Always consult with a healthcare provider before starting any herbal remedy, and ensure that your cancer treatment plan is comprehensive and includes evidence-based medical care.

CHAPTER 4
Mind-Body Practices

Mind-body practices are techniques that harness the connection between mental and physical health, promoting relaxation, reducing stress, and improving overall well-being. In the context of cancer care, these practices can help patients manage symptoms, cope with the emotional and psychological challenges of the disease, and potentially improve treatment outcomes. While mind-body practices are not a substitute for conventional treatments, they can be valuable components of a holistic cancer care plan.

Meditation

Meditation is a practice that involves focusing the mind and eliminating distractions to achieve a state of relaxation, awareness, and inner peace. It has been widely studied for its benefits in reducing stress, anxiety, and depression—common challenges faced by cancer patients.

Potential Benefits: Regular meditation can help reduce stress hormones, improve immune function, and enhance emotional resilience. It may also help manage pain, improve sleep, and reduce fatigue. Some studies suggest that meditation may even have a positive impact on the body's response to cancer treatment.

Techniques: There are various forms of meditation, including mindfulness meditation, guided imagery, and transcendental meditation. Patients can practice meditation on their own or with the help of guided sessions, apps, or classes.

Yoga

Yoga is a mind-body practice that combines physical postures, breathing exercises, and meditation. It is known for its ability to improve flexibility, strength, and balance, but it also offers significant mental and emotional benefits, making it a popular complementary therapy for cancer patients.

Potential Benefits: Yoga can help reduce stress, anxiety, and depression, improve sleep quality, and increase energy levels. It may also help manage pain and improve physical functioning. For cancer patients, gentle yoga practices tailored to their needs can support the healing process and enhance quality of life.

Styles: Different styles of yoga, such as Hatha, Vinyasa, and Restorative yoga, offer varying levels of intensity. Patients should choose a style that suits their physical condition and energy levels, with guidance from a qualified instructor experienced in working with cancer patients.

Acupuncture

Acupuncture is a traditional Chinese medicine practice that involves inserting thin needles into specific points on the body to balance the flow of energy (Qi) and promote healing. It is increasingly used as a complementary therapy in cancer care, particularly for managing symptoms and side effects of treatment.

Potential Benefits: Acupuncture has been shown to be effective in managing chemotherapy-induced nausea and vomiting, reducing pain, and alleviating fatigue. It may also help with anxiety, stress, and sleep disturbances. Some studies suggest that acupuncture can improve overall well-being and quality of life for cancer patients.

Procedure: Acupuncture should be performed by a licensed practitioner who is experienced in treating cancer patients. The practitioner will develop a treatment plan based on the patient's specific symptoms and needs.

Tai Chi and Qigong

Tai Chi and Qigong are ancient Chinese practices that combine gentle physical movements, controlled breathing, and meditation. These practices are designed to enhance the flow of energy in the body, promote relaxation, and improve physical and mental health.

Potential Benefits: Tai Chi and Qigong can help improve balance, flexibility, and strength, while also reducing stress, anxiety, and fatigue. They are particularly beneficial for cancer patients who need gentle exercise that supports both physical and emotional health.

Practice: Both Tai Chi and Qigong can be practiced in groups or individually, with the guidance of an instructor or through videos and online resources. The movements are slow and controlled, making them suitable for people of all ages and fitness levels.

Guided Imagery

Guided imagery involves the use of mental visualization to create calming, positive images and scenarios in the mind. This practice can be a powerful tool for managing stress, reducing anxiety, and promoting relaxation during cancer treatment.

Potential Benefits: Guided imagery can help lower stress hormones, enhance the immune system, and reduce pain and discomfort. It may also help patients feel more in control of their treatment experience and improve their emotional resilience.

Practice: Guided imagery can be practiced with the help of a therapist, through recordings, or independently. Patients are guided to imagine peaceful scenes or scenarios, often accompanied by deep breathing exercises.

Breathing Exercises

Breathing exercises are simple techniques that focus on controlling the breath to reduce stress, calm the mind, and enhance physical relaxation. These exercises are easy to learn and can be practiced anywhere, making them a convenient tool for managing the emotional and physical challenges of cancer.

Potential Benefits: Breathing exercises can help reduce anxiety, improve sleep, lower blood pressure, and enhance overall relaxation. They can also be useful for managing pain and discomfort, particularly during or after cancer treatments.

Techniques: Common breathing exercises include diaphragmatic breathing, box breathing, and the 4-7-8 breathing technique. These exercises typically involve slow, deep breaths, with a focus on the rhythm and depth of breathing.

Art Therapy

Art therapy involves using creative expression, such as drawing, painting, or sculpting, to process emotions, reduce stress, and improve mental health. For cancer patients, art therapy provides a way to explore and express feelings related to their illness in a supportive environment.

Potential Benefits: Art therapy can help reduce stress, anxiety, and depression, improve mood, and provide a sense of accomplishment and self-expression. It can also be a valuable tool for coping with the emotional impact of cancer and its treatments.

Sessions: Art therapy is typically guided by a trained art therapist who helps patients explore their feelings through creative activities. Sessions can be individual or group-based and are tailored to the patient's needs and abilities.

Music Therapy

Music therapy uses music to address physical, emotional, cognitive, and social needs. It can include listening to music, playing instruments, singing, or writing songs. Music therapy is often used in cancer care to improve emotional well-being and manage symptoms.

Potential Benefits: Music therapy can help reduce anxiety, improve mood, and manage pain. It can also provide a sense of comfort and connection, which is particularly important during challenging times.

Sessions: Music therapy sessions are led by a trained music therapist and can be adapted to the patient's preferences and abilities. Sessions may include listening to calming music, engaging in musical activities, or simply enjoying the therapeutic effects of sound.

Mind-body practices offer a holistic approach to supporting cancer patients, addressing the mental, emotional, and physical challenges of the disease. By incorporating these practices into a comprehensive cancer care plan, patients can improve their quality of life, manage symptoms, and foster a sense of well-being. It is important to choose mind-body practices that resonate with individual preferences and needs and to discuss these options with healthcare providers to ensure they complement conventional treatments.

CHAPTER 5

Supplements

Supplements, including vitamins, minerals, and other nutrients, can play a supportive role in cancer care. They may help address nutritional deficiencies, bolster the immune system, and reduce side effects of cancer treatments. However, supplements should be used with caution, as some can interact with conventional cancer therapies or may not be appropriate for all patients. It's essential to consult with a healthcare provider before starting any supplement regimen.

Vitamin D

Vitamin D is essential for bone health, immune function, and overall well-being. Emerging research suggests that adequate levels of vitamin D may also be associated with a lower risk of certain cancers, including breast, prostate, and colorectal cancers. Additionally, vitamin D deficiency is common among cancer patients, particularly those undergoing treatment.

Potential Benefits: Vitamin D may help regulate cell growth, reduce inflammation, and improve immune function. It is also being studied for its potential role in slowing the progression of cancer.

Sources and Dosage: The body naturally produces vitamin D when exposed to sunlight, but supplementation may be necessary for those with low levels, especially in regions with limited sunlight. Vitamin D supplements are available in various forms, including vitamin D2 (ergocalciferol) and vitamin D3 (cholecalciferol). A healthcare provider can recommend the appropriate dosage based on individual needs.

Omega-3 Fatty Acids

Omega-3 fatty acids, found in fish oil and certain plant oils, are known for their anti-inflammatory properties and are essential for heart and brain health. They may also have a role in cancer prevention and management by reducing inflammation, which is linked to cancer progression.

Potential Benefits: Omega-3s may help reduce cancer-related inflammation, improve immune response, and potentially enhance the effectiveness of certain cancer treatments. They are also beneficial for cardiovascular health, which is important for cancer patients at risk of heart disease.

Sources and Dosage: Omega-3s are found in fatty fish like salmon, mackerel, and sardines, as well as in flaxseeds, chia seeds, and walnuts. Fish oil supplements are a common source of omega-3s. The recommended dosage varies, so it's best to consult with a healthcare provider.

Probiotics

Probiotics are live microorganisms that support a healthy gut microbiome, which is crucial for overall health and immune function. A balanced gut microbiome can help the body better handle cancer treatments and may reduce gastrointestinal side effects such as diarrhea and constipation.

Potential Benefits: Probiotics may help restore gut flora balance, reduce inflammation, and improve digestion during cancer treatment. Some studies suggest that a healthy gut microbiome can support the immune system and potentially improve treatment outcomes.

Sources and Dosage: Probiotics are found in fermented foods like yogurt, kefir, sauerkraut, and kimchi. They are also available in supplement form, with various strains offering different benefits. It's important to choose a high-quality probiotic and follow dosage recommendations from a healthcare provider.

Curcumin

Curcumin, the active compound in turmeric, has been extensively studied for its anti-inflammatory and anti-cancer properties. As a supplement, curcumin may help inhibit cancer cell growth, reduce inflammation, and enhance the effectiveness of conventional cancer treatments.

Potential Benefits: Curcumin has been shown to interfere with cancer cell signaling pathways, potentially slowing cancer progression and making cancer cells more susceptible to treatment. It may also help manage inflammation and oxidative stress in the body.

Sources and Dosage: Curcumin supplements are available in various forms, including capsules, tablets, and powders. Because curcumin is poorly absorbed on its own, supplements often include piperine (from black pepper) or other compounds to enhance bioavailability. The appropriate dosage should be determined by a healthcare provider.

Vitamin C
Vitamin C is a powerful antioxidant that supports immune function and may help protect against cancer by neutralizing free radicals. High-dose vitamin C, administered intravenously, has been explored as a complementary therapy in cancer treatment, though its efficacy is still under investigation.

Potential Benefits: Vitamin C may help boost the immune system, reduce inflammation, and protect cells from damage during cancer treatment. Some studies suggest that high-dose intravenous vitamin C may improve quality of life and reduce the side effects of chemotherapy.

Sources and Dosage: Vitamin C is abundant in fruits and vegetables, particularly citrus fruits, strawberries, bell peppers, and broccoli. Oral supplements are available, but the high doses used in some cancer therapies require intravenous administration, which should only be done under medical supervision.

Zinc

Zinc is an essential mineral involved in immune function, wound healing, and DNA synthesis. It plays a critical role in maintaining a healthy immune system, which is particularly important for cancer patients undergoing treatment.

Potential Benefits: Zinc may help support immune function, reduce inflammation, and promote healing. It is also important for taste and smell, which can be affected by cancer treatments. Zinc supplementation may help alleviate these sensory changes.

Sources and Dosage: Zinc is found in foods like meat, shellfish, legumes, seeds, and nuts. Supplements are available in various forms, including zinc gluconate, zinc sulfate, and zinc citrate. The appropriate dosage should be based on individual needs and determined by a healthcare provider.

Melatonin

Melatonin is a hormone that regulates sleep-wake cycles and has antioxidant properties. It is often used as a supplement to help with sleep disturbances, which are common among cancer patients. Emerging research also suggests that melatonin may have anti-cancer effects.

Potential Benefits: Melatonin may improve sleep quality, reduce anxiety, and help manage symptoms like fatigue. Some studies suggest that melatonin may enhance the effectiveness of certain cancer treatments and protect healthy cells from radiation damage.

Sources and Dosage: Melatonin supplements are available in various dosages, typically taken in the evening to promote sleep. The dosage should be personalized based on individual needs and discussed with a healthcare provider.

Green Tea Extract

Green tea extract is rich in polyphenols, particularly epigallocatechin gallate (EGCG), which have potent antioxidant and anti-cancer properties. Green tea extract is often used as a supplement to support overall health and may play a role in cancer prevention and management.

Potential Benefits: EGCG has been shown to inhibit cancer cell growth, reduce inflammation, and protect against DNA damage. Green tea extract supplements may help support immune function and complement conventional cancer treatments.

Sources and Dosage: Green tea extract is available in capsules, tablets, and liquid forms. It's important to choose a supplement that provides a standardized dose of EGCG. Dosage should be guided by a healthcare provider.

While supplements can provide valuable support in cancer care, they should be used thoughtfully and under the guidance of a healthcare provider. The effectiveness and safety of supplements can vary depending on the individual's overall health, type of cancer, and current treatments. It's essential to integrate supplements as part of a comprehensive cancer care plan that includes evidence-based medical treatments, a nutritious diet, regular physical activity, and mind-body practices.

CHAPTER 6

Lifestyle Changes

Lifestyle changes play a crucial role in supporting cancer treatment and improving overall well-being. By adopting healthier habits, cancer patients can enhance their quality of life, reduce treatment side effects, and possibly lower the risk of cancer recurrence. These changes should be personalized to fit individual needs and preferences, and they can complement medical treatments in a holistic approach to cancer care.

Healthy Diet

Maintaining a balanced and nutritious diet is vital for cancer patients. Proper nutrition supports the immune system, helps manage treatment side effects, and provides the energy needed to cope with the physical and emotional demands of cancer treatment.

Plant-Based Diet: Emphasizing a diet rich in fruits, vegetables, whole grains, nuts, and seeds provides essential vitamins, minerals, antioxidants, and fiber. These foods can help reduce inflammation and support the body's natural defenses against cancer.

Protein: Adequate protein intake is important for healing and maintaining muscle mass, especially during treatment. Lean sources of protein include poultry, fish, legumes, tofu, and dairy products.

Hydration: Staying well-hydrated is crucial, particularly during chemotherapy or radiation therapy, which can cause dehydration. Water, herbal teas, and broths are good options.

Avoiding Processed Foods: Limiting the intake of processed foods, sugary drinks, and red or processed meats can help reduce the risk of inflammation and other health complications.

Regular Physical Activity

Regular exercise is beneficial for cancer patients at all stages of the disease. It can improve physical strength, reduce fatigue, and enhance mental health. Exercise also supports the immune system and may help reduce the risk of cancer recurrence.

Types of Exercise: Aerobic exercises like walking, swimming, or cycling, along with strength training and flexibility exercises, are all beneficial. Yoga and tai chi are also excellent for combining physical activity with stress reduction.

Personalized Exercise Plan: The type and intensity of exercise should be tailored to the individual's health status, treatment phase, and physical capabilities. Consulting with a healthcare provider or physical therapist is advisable to develop a safe and effective exercise plan.

Consistency: Even small amounts of regular physical activity can make a significant difference. The key is to remain consistent and to choose activities that are enjoyable and sustainable.
Stress Management

Managing stress is essential for overall health and well-being, especially for cancer patients. Chronic stress can weaken the immune system and exacerbate symptoms, making it important to find effective ways to relax and maintain emotional balance.

Mindfulness and Meditation: Practicing mindfulness, meditation, or deep breathing exercises can help reduce stress and anxiety. These practices encourage relaxation and a sense of calm, which can be particularly beneficial during treatment.

Time in Nature: Spending time outdoors in natural settings can have a calming effect and improve mood. Activities like walking in a park, gardening, or simply sitting in a peaceful outdoor space can help reduce stress.

Counseling and Support Groups: Talking to a therapist, counselor, or participating in a support group can provide emotional support and coping strategies. It's important to address the emotional impact of cancer and seek help when needed.

Adequate Sleep

Quality sleep is crucial for healing and recovery, yet many cancer patients struggle with sleep disturbances due to pain, anxiety, or treatment side effects. Ensuring adequate rest is important for maintaining physical and mental health.

Sleep Hygiene: Establishing a regular sleep routine, creating a comfortable sleep environment, and avoiding stimulants like caffeine before bed can improve sleep quality.
Relaxation Techniques: Practices such as deep breathing, progressive muscle relaxation, or guided imagery can help relax the body and mind, making it easier to fall asleep.

Addressing Sleep Issues: If sleep problems persist, it may be helpful to speak with a healthcare provider about possible solutions, such as cognitive behavioral therapy for insomnia (CBT-I) or other interventions.

Avoiding Tobacco and Alcohol

Avoiding tobacco and limiting alcohol consumption are critical lifestyle changes for cancer patients. Both substances are linked to an increased risk of cancer and can interfere with the effectiveness of treatment.

Tobacco: Smoking or using tobacco products can worsen the prognosis for cancer patients and increase the risk of secondary cancers. Quitting smoking is one of the most important steps a cancer patient can take for their health.

Alcohol: Alcohol can interfere with certain cancer treatments and may increase the risk of recurrence. Limiting alcohol intake, or abstaining altogether, can support overall health and recovery.

Maintaining a Healthy Weight

Achieving and maintaining a healthy weight is important for reducing the risk of cancer recurrence and improving overall health. Weight management can also help alleviate treatment-related side effects and support a better prognosis.

Balanced Diet and Exercise: A combination of a balanced diet and regular physical activity is key to maintaining a healthy weight. This includes portion control, mindful eating, and staying active.

Professional Support: For those struggling with weight management, seeking advice from a dietitian or nutritionist who specializes in oncology can provide personalized guidance and support.
Limiting Exposure to Environmental Toxins

Reducing exposure to environmental toxins, such as certain chemicals, pesticides, and pollutants, can contribute to better health and may reduce the risk of cancer recurrence.

Household Products: Choose natural or non-toxic cleaning and personal care products to minimize exposure to harmful chemicals.

Dietary Choices: Opting for organic foods, when possible, can reduce exposure to pesticides and other chemicals.

Air Quality: Improving indoor air quality by using air purifiers, ventilating living spaces, and avoiding the use of products that release harmful fumes can also be beneficial.

Building Strong Relationships

Social support is a powerful tool in cancer care. Building and maintaining strong relationships with family, friends, and support groups can provide emotional strength, reduce feelings of isolation, and improve overall quality of life.

Connecting with Others: Engaging in meaningful conversations, participating in social activities, and reaching out for help when needed can strengthen bonds and provide much-needed support.

Support Groups: Joining a cancer support group, either in-person or online, allows patients to connect with others who are experiencing similar challenges, providing a sense of community and understanding.

Lifestyle changes are an essential component of a holistic approach to cancer care. By adopting healthier habits, cancer patients can support their treatment, improve their quality of life, and potentially reduce the risk of cancer recurrence. These changes should be personalized to each individual's needs and preferences, and they should be integrated into a comprehensive cancer care plan that includes medical treatments, nutritional support, mind-body practices, and regular follow-ups with healthcare providers.

CHAPTER 7

Supportive Therapies

Supportive therapies encompass a range of treatments and interventions designed to help cancer patients manage symptoms, reduce side effects, and improve their overall quality of life. These therapies do not aim to cure cancer but provide relief from the physical, emotional, and psychological challenges associated with the disease and its treatment. Integrating supportive therapies into cancer care can help patients cope more effectively and maintain a better quality of life throughout their treatment journey.

Pain Management

Pain is a common and often debilitating symptom for many cancer patients. Effective pain management is essential for improving quality of life and ensuring that patients can continue with their daily activities and treatments.

Medications: Pain management often involves the use of analgesics, including non-steroidal anti-inflammatory drugs (NSAIDs), acetaminophen, and opioids. The choice of medication depends on the severity of the pain and the patient's overall health.

Nerve Blocks and Epidural Injections: For certain types of cancer-related pain, nerve blocks or epidural injections may be used to interrupt pain signals and provide relief.

Complementary Approaches: Integrating complementary therapies such as acupuncture, massage, and relaxation techniques can enhance pain relief and reduce the need for high doses of medication.

Palliative Care

Palliative care focuses on providing relief from the symptoms, pain, and stress of serious illness, including cancer. It is appropriate at any stage of cancer and can be provided alongside curative treatment.

Comprehensive Support: Palliative care addresses not only physical symptoms but also emotional, social, and spiritual needs. It involves a multidisciplinary team that may include doctors, nurses, social workers, and chaplains.

Symptom Management: In addition to pain management, palliative care can help manage symptoms like nausea, vomiting, fatigue, shortness of breath, and depression.

Communication and Decision-Making: Palliative care providers also assist patients and their families in making informed decisions about treatment options and end-of-life care, ensuring that care aligns with the patient's values and preferences.

Lymphedema Therapy
Lymphedema is a condition characterized by swelling, typically in the arms or legs, caused by a build-up of lymph fluid. It is a common side effect of cancer treatments that involve the removal of lymph nodes, such as surgery for breast cancer.

Manual Lymphatic Drainage (MLD): MLD is a specialized massage technique that helps stimulate the flow of lymph fluid and reduce swelling. It should be performed by a certified lymphedema therapist.

Compression Garments: Wearing compression sleeves or stockings can help manage lymphedema by promoting fluid circulation and reducing swelling.

Exercise: Gentle, low-impact exercises, such as swimming or walking, can improve lymphatic flow and prevent worsening of lymphedema.

Nutritional Support
Nutritional support is crucial for cancer patients, especially those who experience appetite loss, weight loss, or difficulty eating due to treatment side effects. Proper nutrition helps maintain strength, supports the immune system, and improves overall well-being.

Dietary Counseling: A registered dietitian who specializes in oncology can provide personalized nutrition advice, helping patients manage symptoms like nausea, taste changes, and swallowing difficulties.

Oral Nutritional Supplements: For patients who have trouble eating enough food, high-calorie and high-protein oral supplements can provide essential nutrients.

Tube Feeding: In some cases, when oral intake is insufficient, enteral nutrition (tube feeding) may be necessary to ensure adequate nutritional support.

Psychological Support
The psychological impact of cancer can be profound, leading to feelings of anxiety, depression, fear, and uncertainty. Psychological support helps patients cope with these emotions and improves their mental health during and after treatment.

Counseling and Therapy: Individual or group therapy with a psychologist or counselor can help patients address emotional challenges, develop coping strategies, and reduce stress. Cognitive-behavioral therapy (CBT) is particularly effective in managing anxiety and depression.

Support Groups: Joining a cancer support group allows patients to connect with others who are facing similar challenges, providing a sense of community and shared understanding.

Mindfulness and Relaxation Techniques: Practices such as mindfulness meditation, guided imagery, and relaxation exercises can reduce stress and improve emotional well-being.

Physical Therapy and Rehabilitation
Cancer treatments can lead to physical impairments, such as reduced mobility, muscle weakness, and fatigue. Physical therapy and rehabilitation help patients regain strength, improve mobility, and maintain independence.

Exercise Programs: A physical therapist can design a personalized exercise program to improve strength, flexibility, and endurance, helping patients recover from surgery or cope with treatment-related fatigue.

Occupational Therapy: Occupational therapy focuses on helping patients perform daily activities, such as dressing, bathing, and cooking, despite physical limitations. Therapists may also recommend adaptive devices to improve independence.

Lymphedema Management: Physical therapists trained in lymphedema management can provide exercises and treatments to reduce swelling and improve lymphatic circulation.
Integrative Oncology

Integrative oncology combines conventional cancer treatments with complementary therapies to support the whole person—body, mind, and spirit. This approach aims to reduce treatment side effects, improve quality of life, and enhance overall well-being.

Acupuncture: Acupuncture can help manage treatment-related side effects such as pain, nausea, and fatigue. It is particularly effective in reducing chemotherapy-induced nausea and vomiting.

Massage Therapy: Massage therapy provides relief from pain, anxiety, and stress. It can also improve circulation and reduce muscle tension, enhancing overall comfort and relaxation.

Herbal Medicine: Certain herbs and botanical supplements may help support the immune system, reduce inflammation, and alleviate symptoms. However, it is important to consult with a healthcare provider before using any herbal remedies to avoid potential interactions with cancer treatments.

Spiritual Care

Spiritual care addresses the existential and spiritual concerns that may arise during a cancer diagnosis. It helps patients find meaning, purpose, and peace, regardless of their religious or spiritual beliefs.

Chaplaincy Services: Chaplains provide spiritual support, offering a listening ear and guidance on spiritual matters. They can also assist with religious rituals and practices if desired.

Mind-Body Practices: Meditation, prayer, and mindfulness practices can help patients connect with their inner selves and find spiritual comfort during challenging times.

Supportive Conversations: Engaging in conversations about spirituality, meaning, and purpose with a trusted counselor or spiritual advisor can provide a sense of peace and acceptance.

Sleep Therapy

Sleep disturbances are common among cancer patients due to pain, anxiety, and treatment side effects. Addressing sleep issues is important for overall health and recovery.

Cognitive Behavioral Therapy for Insomnia (CBT-I): CBT-I is a structured program that helps patients address the thoughts and behaviors that contribute to sleep problems, improving sleep quality over time.

Sleep Hygiene: Good sleep hygiene practices, such as maintaining a regular sleep schedule, creating a comfortable sleep environment, and limiting caffeine intake, can promote better sleep.

Medications: In some cases, medications may be prescribed to help with sleep, but these should be used under the guidance of a healthcare provider.

Supportive therapies are an integral part of comprehensive cancer care. They help manage symptoms, reduce side effects, and improve the quality of life for cancer patients. By addressing the physical, emotional, and psychological aspects of cancer, these therapies support patients throughout their treatment journey, helping them cope more effectively and maintain a better quality of life. It is important for patients to work closely with their healthcare team to identify the most appropriate supportive therapies based on their individual needs and treatment goals.

CHAPTER 8

Important Considerations

When integrating natural remedies, supportive therapies, and lifestyle changes into cancer care, several key considerations should be taken into account to ensure safety, effectiveness, and alignment with conventional treatments. Here are some important factors to keep in mind:

Consult with Healthcare Providers

Professional Guidance: Always consult with oncologists and other healthcare professionals before starting any new therapies, supplements, or significant lifestyle changes. This ensures that any new approach is safe and compatible with current cancer treatments.

Interdisciplinary Care: Work with a multidisciplinary team that may include oncologists, nutritionists, physical therapists, and mental health professionals to develop a comprehensive and coordinated care plan.

Evidence-Based Practices

Scientific Research: Prioritize therapies and supplements that are supported by credible scientific research and clinical evidence. Be cautious with remedies that lack robust evidence or that are promoted based on anecdotal claims alone.

Ongoing Research: Stay informed about emerging research and developments in cancer care.

Evidence-based practices can evolve as new studies are published and treatment options are updated.

Potential Interactions

Drug Interactions: Some natural remedies, supplements, and herbal products can interact with conventional cancer treatments, potentially affecting their efficacy or causing adverse effects. Always disclose all supplements and therapies to your healthcare team.

Side Effects: Be aware of potential side effects of both conventional treatments and supportive therapies. Monitor any new symptoms or changes and report them to your healthcare provider.

Personalization

Individual Needs: Treatment and supportive care should be personalized based on the individual's type of cancer, stage of disease, overall health, and treatment plan. What works for one person may not be suitable for another.

Customization: Tailor lifestyle changes, dietary adjustments, and supportive therapies to fit personal preferences, cultural practices, and specific health conditions.

Safety and Quality

Quality Control: Choose high-quality supplements and natural products from reputable sources. Look for products that have been tested for purity and potency.

Safety Standards: Ensure that any complementary therapies, such as acupuncture or massage, are provided by certified and experienced practitioners who follow established safety standards.

Communication and Coordination

Open Dialogue: Maintain open communication with your healthcare team about all aspects of your care, including the use of natural remedies and supportive therapies. This helps ensure coordinated care and avoids potential conflicts between different treatment modalities.

Documentation: Keep detailed records of all treatments, supplements, and therapies used. This information can be valuable for your healthcare team in monitoring progress and managing any issues that arise.

Emotional and Psychological Support

Mental Health: Recognize the importance of addressing emotional and psychological needs alongside physical treatments. Incorporate strategies for managing stress, anxiety, and depression as part of your overall care plan.

Support Networks: Engage with support groups, counseling services, and other resources that provide emotional and social support during the cancer journey.

Realistic Expectations

Understand Limitations: Be aware that while supportive therapies and lifestyle changes can enhance quality of life and help manage symptoms, they are not a substitute for conventional cancer treatments. They should be viewed as complementary rather than curative.

Set Goals: Set realistic and achievable goals for incorporating natural remedies and supportive therapies into your care plan. Focus on improvements in quality of life and symptom management rather than seeking a cure.

Holistic Approach

Comprehensive Care: Adopt a holistic approach that considers the whole person—body, mind, and spirit. Integrate supportive therapies, lifestyle changes, and conventional treatments in a way that supports overall well-being.

Balance: Strive for a balance between conventional treatments and complementary approaches to maximize the benefits of both and ensure comprehensive care.

Monitoring and Evaluation

Regular Check-Ups: Schedule regular follow-up appointments with your healthcare team to monitor the effects of any new therapies or lifestyle changes on your overall health and cancer treatment.

Adjustments: Be prepared to adjust your care plan based on ongoing evaluations and feedback from your healthcare team. Flexibility and adaptability are key to effective cancer management.

Integrating natural remedies, supportive therapies, and lifestyle changes into cancer care requires careful consideration and collaboration with healthcare professionals. By focusing on evidence-based practices, ensuring safety, personalizing care, and maintaining open communication, patients can enhance their overall well-being and support their cancer treatment journey.

CHAPTER 9

Conclusion

Integrating natural remedies, supportive therapies, and lifestyle changes into cancer care represents a comprehensive approach to enhancing the quality of life for individuals undergoing treatment. By combining conventional medical treatments with complementary strategies, patients can manage symptoms more effectively, reduce side effects, and improve their overall well-being.

Key Takeaways:

Holistic Care: A holistic approach that addresses the physical, emotional, and psychological aspects of cancer is crucial. This includes integrating evidence-based natural remedies, supportive therapies, and healthy lifestyle practices alongside conventional treatments.

Professional Guidance: Consulting with healthcare providers is essential to ensure that any new therapies or lifestyle changes are safe and appropriate for each individual's specific cancer diagnosis and treatment plan. Open communication with the healthcare team helps avoid potential interactions and supports coordinated care.

Personalization: Treatment and supportive care should be tailored to meet the unique needs and preferences of each patient. Personalized care plans enhance the effectiveness of interventions and improve overall quality of life.

Safety and Quality: Emphasizing the use of high-quality supplements, reputable practitioners, and evidence-based practices helps ensure the safety and effectiveness of complementary therapies. Monitoring for side effects and interactions is also vital.

Emotional Support: Addressing emotional and psychological needs through counseling, support groups, and stress management techniques is an integral part of cancer care. Emotional well-being significantly impacts physical health and treatment outcomes.

Realistic Expectations: While natural remedies and supportive therapies can offer significant benefits, they should be viewed as complementary rather than curative. Balancing expectations and focusing on improvements in quality of life and symptom management is essential.

Ongoing Evaluation: Regular follow-ups with healthcare providers and ongoing evaluation of the care plan ensure that interventions remain effective and adjustments are made as needed. Flexibility and adaptability are key to successful cancer management.

In summary, a thoughtful and coordinated approach to incorporating natural remedies, supportive therapies, and lifestyle changes can enhance cancer care and support patients throughout their treatment journey. By focusing on a comprehensive and individualized plan, patients can achieve better outcomes, manage symptoms effectively, and improve their overall quality of life.